DEC 11

P9-BYF-373

EPIDEMICS AND SOCIETY™

POLIO

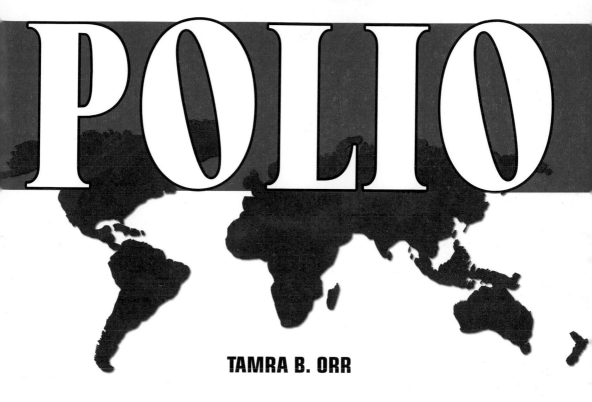

TAMRA B. ORR

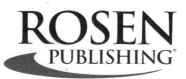

ROSEN
PUBLISHING®

New York

Published in 2011 by The Rosen Publishing Group, Inc.
29 East 21st Street, New York, NY 10010

First Edition

Library of Congress Cataloging-in-Publication Data

Orr, Tamra.
Polio / Tamra B. Orr.—1st ed.
     p. cm.—(Epidemics and society)
Includes bibliographical references and index.
ISBN 978-1-4358-9436-5 (lib. bdg.)
1. Poliomyelitis—Popular works. I. Title.
RC180.2.O77 2011
616.8'35—dc22

                                                                        2009045562

Manufactured in the United States of America

CPSIA Compliance Information: Batch #S10YA: For further information, contact Rosen Publishing, New York, New York, at 1-800-237-9932.

On the cover: This is a digital illustration of the microscopic poliovirus.

CONTENTS

The history of medicine is full of stories that detail exactly how microscopic bacteria and even tinier viruses somehow snuck their way into the places where humans lived, worked, and played. Without warning, like small, silent armies, they spread out, leaping from person to person. They began attacking the human body, doling out pain, sickness, and death as they went. For years, these invaders won each battle because no one knew how to strike back. Where were the attacks coming from? What weapons did the disease use, and how could they be overcome? What was the enemy's weakness—or did it even have one?

One of these miniature armies, the poliomyelitis virus, terrified, crippled, and killed people

4

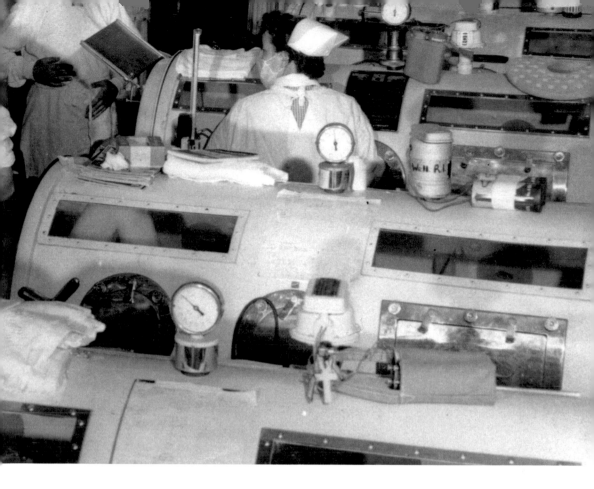

Hospitals were often overwhelmed with emergency polio patients. Trying to make room for them, as well as for the bulky iron lungs, was a complicated and chaotic task for the staff.

for thousands of years, without being discovered or halted. Like the agents (causes) of other infectious diseases before it, the poliovirus arrived concealed inside the most innocent and basic of human needs: water.

Outbreaks of polio had most likely been appearing for centuries. But it was not until the late eighteenth century that a doctor gave the illness a name and attempted to classify it. Since then, the disease—and the virus that causes it—has gone through many different names. In the end, it has come to be known as poliomyelitis, or polio, for short.

CHAPTER ONE

A SILENT ARMY

The word "poliomyelitis" combines "gray" (Greek *polios*), "marrow" (Greek *myelos*), and "infection" or "inflammation" (Latin *itis*). Put it all together and it translates into "the inflammation of the gray matter of the spinal cord."

Like some other infectious diseases, polio is caused by infection with a tiny, microscopic virus. Although it is small, the poliovirus can be quite powerful. It is also quite complicated because this tiny virus comes in three types. And within those three types are many sub-strains. It is little wonder that polio confused and confounded scientists and doctors for so many years.

How the Enemy Gains Entry

To understand how the poliovirus works, let's look at how it got to people in the first place. The virus is waterborne. When traces of fecal matter (solid waste) from someone infected with the poliovirus were found in the water, it meant the virus could be there as well. Anyone who swam in or drank the contaminated water, or had contact with someone or something that had touched the water, was at risk for contracting the poliovirus.

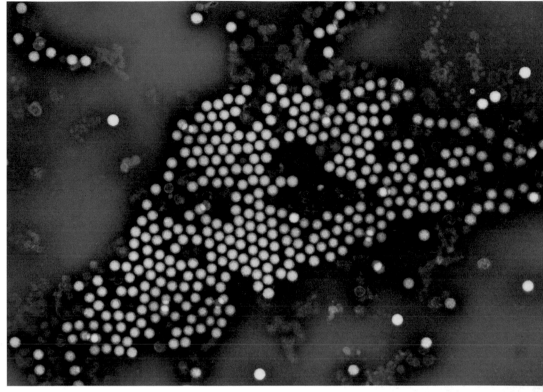

This cluster of polio virus particles shows how each one is made of an outer protein coat surrounding a core of genetic material. It is hard to believe something so tiny could be so devastating to so many people.

Water had long been a culprit in spreading disease. During the Industrial Revolution (1750–1850), the United States experienced enormous changes. Life on the farm increasingly gave way to jobs in factories. People began to stream out of the country and crowd into cities to find work. Too many people and not enough development of sanitation systems resulted in sewage problems in urban areas. Waste was often tossed out the window onto the street or into the closest pond or other body of water. Viruses and bacteria from human waste were spread through this water and often infected people when they drank the water.

In these rapidly growing cities of the eighteenth and nineteenth centuries, water supplies were quickly contaminated with waste products from homes and factories. Lakes, rivers, reservoirs, and wells were turned into the perfect breeding grounds for disease. The infectious agents that caused typhoid fever and cholera were both spread through water and killed countless people.

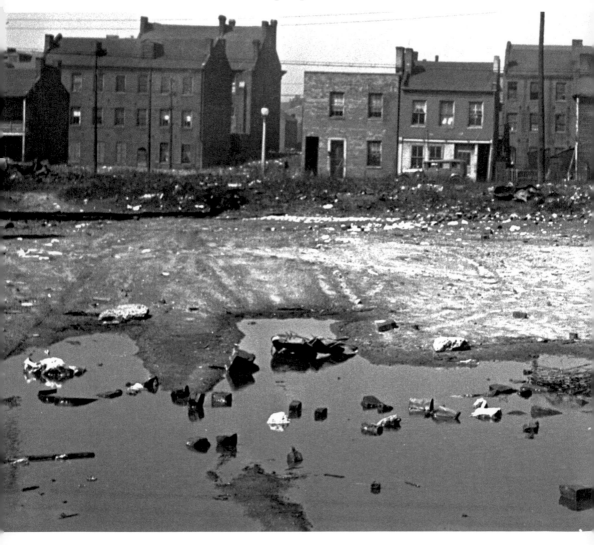

Playing outside in lakes, ponds, and even puddles was just another fun thing to do for young children. There was little way of knowing that the water could be the source of a terrible and sometimes crippling or even fatal disease.

Hiding among all of the other bacteria and viruses was the poliovirus. People had been exposed to it for years. As a result, most of them built up natural immunities to it. Babies were protected by the antibodies passed to them from their mothers. Ironically, all of that changed when sanitation systems were developed. Water was now treated and made cleaner. As a consequence, exposure to the poliovirus dropped dramatically. Girls who grew up in this era of increasing sanitation eventually became mothers, but they no longer had the antibodies to pass on to their babies for protection. No one had the chance to build up immunity to polio anymore.

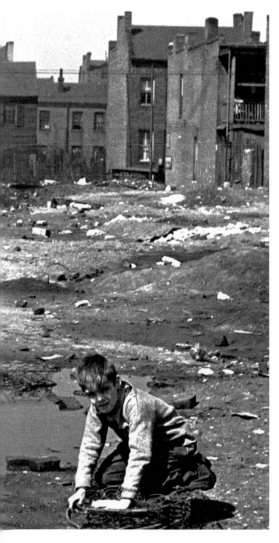

Now, when people forgot to wash their hands after changing a diaper or going to the bathroom, or swam in water with someone who didn't wash properly, or touched something a contaminated person had touched, they were at risk of contracting the virus. Polio began to attack the youngest part of the population—and it often attacked very hard.

The poliovirus typically followed the following infection pathway inside the body:

- Enter through the mouth.
- Multiply in the throat and then the gastrointestinal tract.
- Move into the bloodstream.

In the relatively rare cases of paralytic polio, the virus would then shift to the central nervous system, replicate (make copies of itself), and destroy motor neuron cells (resulting in paralysis).

Types of Polio Infection

Although this was the disease process identified by doctors, the poliovirus was tricky and unpredictable and did not affect everyone the same way. Instead, it presented itself in four different ways:

1. Asymptomatic

The person who has this type of infection may never even realize he or she is sick. It is the mildest form, and most people do not experience any symptoms. The vast majority of the people exposed to the poliovirus had an asymptomatic infection.

2. Abortive

This type of infection with the poliovirus is noticeable but not much more troublesome than asymptomatic infection. A person might feel more tired than usual, with perhaps a headache, sore throat, or fever. It may feel like little more than the common cold. Sometimes extra symptoms include intestinal problems like vomiting, pain, constipation, or diarrhea.

3. Non-paralytic

This type of polio illness is more serious because the poliovirus has reached the spinal cord, so the victim has all of the above symptoms but also a stiff neck and achy, sore limbs. However, those with non-paralytic illness usually recover.

4. Paralytic

By far, the worst type of polio is this one. In these cases, the virus has actually arrived at the central nervous system and launched an attack against the vulnerable motor neurons found there. Motor neurons have an extremely important function: It is their job to pass messages and instructions from the brain to the muscles. These messages and instructions tell the muscles how and when to move. If the messages cannot get through, communication is lost. Muscles are still. The person is paralyzed. Sensation is still there. The muscles still hurt, but the ability to control them is gone. In this form of polio, the leg muscles are often the first ones affected, followed by the arms and trunk and, worst of all, the muscles used for breathing. Less than 1 percent of the people who were infected by the poliovirus had the paralytic type—but that still translated to thousands of victims.

Those that were diagnosed with the paralytic form of polio were often further subdivided into distinct groups, depending on what set of motor neurons were affected the most. Those in the spinal group, for example, dealt with the effects of damage to the nerve cells of the spinal cord, chest, arms, and legs. The bulbar group struggled with the results of polio attacking the nerve cells of their brainstems, where the cranial nerves are. An attack here might interfere with a person's ability to hear, see, smell, taste, or swallow. It was often fatal. The bulbospinal group dealt with both spinal and cranial complications, as well as problems with heart function.

Wild Theories

With every new outbreak of polio, people looked for someone or something to blame for what was happening. They looked in logical directions—and some that were not so logical. Some of the incorrect disease and infection theories that were circulating included:

- Immigrants from one country or another brought the disease with them.
- Wild animals or even pets were to blame, resulting in the useless extermination of thousands of rats, mice, stray dogs and cats, and even house pets.
- Insect bites carried the poliovirus—either mosquitoes or flies. As a result, streets were fogged with toxic pesticides and insecticides like DDT.
- The nerve gases used in Europe during World War I had drifted across the Atlantic Ocean to the United States and made people sick.
- Tarantulas carried in on imported bananas injected the poliovirus into the fruit.
- The poliovirus was hidden in ice cream, soda, or candy.
- Radio waves carried the poliovirus.
- Only those with certain skin colors, face shapes, postures, or teeth positioning were affected by the disease.

Tracking the Virus Through History

No one knows when the poliovirus might have first appeared in a drop of water. Experts suspect, however, that it might have been as far back as the time of ancient Egypt. A three-thousand-year-old stone engraving shows a man with a withered leg, leaning on a staff for support. Was it polio that caused this deformity? The man's affliction remains a mystery.

It wasn't until 1789 that the very first clinical description of polio appeared in print. It was identified by a British physician named Michael Underwood. He had noticed an odd disease that apparently affected young children, sometimes leaving them unable to walk or move. He attributed the problem, however, to "teething and foul bowels," not a virus (bacteria and viruses had not yet been discovered or understood).

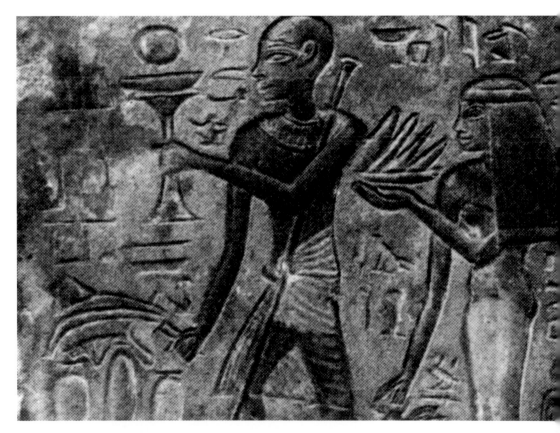

Dating to 1500 BCE, this Egyptian engraving of a man with a withered leg and a staff for support gives scientists clues that polio may have existed for thousands of years.

Next, a German orthope-
dist, Dr. Jacob von Heine, wrote
of a strange "infantile paralysis" and detailed how it
appeared to target the spinal
cord. More than fifty years later,
Dr. Ivar Wickman, one of
Heine's students, discovered
even more about the way this
disease spread. The idea that it
was contagious was already
accepted. But it was Wickman
who figured out that it was not
just the seriously affected
patients who could spread the
disease, but also the ones who
had only mild symptoms. They
were just as contagious.

By 1908, two Austrian
doctors, Karl Landsteiner and
Erwin Popper, were able to
identify the poliovirus for the
first time. The first reportable
epidemic of the disease had
already occurred more than a
dozen years earlier in Vermont, but, in 1916, another one
broke out. During this latest epidemic, the victims numbered
into the thousands. People were getting desperate for
answers—but they were even more desperate for a cure.

A cure would still be several years off, however. Instead,
rumors, fear, mistaken theories, and misguided treatments
would continue to be the order of the day. More children

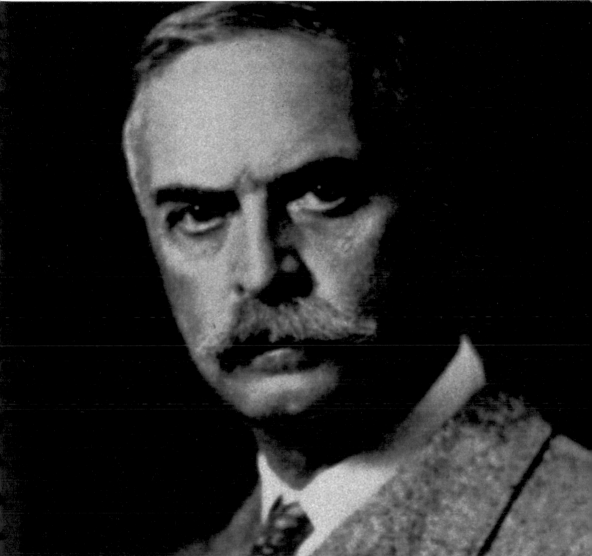

Karl Landsteiner was one of the many physicians who worked to track down evidence about the mysterious polio disease and figure out what could be done to fight it before it claimed any more victims.

would become sick. Many would become crippled. Some would even become paralyzed and die. Polio continued to cut a grim swath of destruction. Hope and salvation were still a long way off.

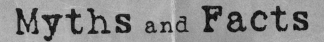

Myths and Facts

MYTH Only children can become infected by the poliovirus and become ill.

FACT Polio can strike at any age, but it mainly affects children under the age of five. Half of all cases involve children under the age of three. Yet unimmunized people of all ages can be infected by the poliovirus. In the past, polio outbreaks occurred mainly in children and adolescents because many older people had already been exposed to the virus and had developed immunity. Unvaccinated adults are unlikely to develop polio in North America because the risk of encountering the virus is so low nowadays. Yet if unvaccinated children or adults are planning to travel to a country where the virus is still active, they are strongly encouraged to receive the vaccine.

MYTH Everyone who gets infected by the poliovirus becomes paralyzed.

FACT Less than 1 percent of polio infections result in paralysis that is either temporary or permanent. Only one in two hundred infections lead to irreversible paralysis. Of patients who experience paralysis, 5 to 10 percent die when the muscles needed for breathing are affected.

MYTH Polio has been "cured" and eradicated.

FACT There is no cure for polio. It can only be prevented through vaccination. Multiple vaccinations throughout the early years of a child's life will provide him or her with lifelong immunity. Polio has not been eradicated worldwide. It is still endemic (found regularly and commonly) in seven countries, especially where sanitation systems are poor. Of all global cases, 98 percent are found in India, Nigeria, and Pakistan.

ATTACKING CITIES AND A NATION'S LEADER

The silent army that was the poliovirus arrived in parts of Europe in the early nineteenth century. A few years later, it had marched across the Atlantic Ocean to attack communities throughout the United States. Each time a town or city was hit, doctors learned a little bit more about the poliovirus and how it operated.

In 1887, Swedish pediatrician Karl Oscar Medin noted that patients typically suffered through two fevers, and the paralysis did not appear until after the second one. The early theory that polio was caused by a virus that multiplied in the lungs slowly gave way to evidence that it reproduced in the digestive tract instead. Scientists and physicians experimented on rabbits, mice, guinea pigs, and monkeys in an attempt to learn more about how the virus operated.

New York City Besieged

Outbreaks popped up in Mason City, Iowa; Cincinnati, Ohio; and Buffalo, New York. In the summer of 1916, New York City was hit, and fear began to grow in earnest. In the borough of

Brooklyn, a few children woke up unable to move. Parents rushed them to the hospital only to find doctors as baffled as they were.

In the beginning, many people placed blame on the large number of Italian immigrants living in the area. Could these people have somehow brought the disease with them from the old country? It was a baseless, misguided fear; Italian immigrants were not the cause of this mysterious disease outbreak. It took weeks before physicians realized what they were facing: a polio epidemic. As the disease spread throughout the city's other four densely populated boroughs— Manhattan, Queens, the Bronx, and Staten Island—New York families began to panic.

As the months went by and patients kept flowing into the city's hospitals, the roads out of New York became flooded with people trying to escape to the country, where they hoped it would be safer. Train stations were swamped, and every departing train was jam-packed. As people fought to get away, they were unwittingly spreading the disease as they went. Ignorant of how the disease was actually spread, New York

City mayor John P. Mitchell ordered the streets cleaned and garbage disposed of immediately in the hopes that it would make a difference. It didn't. He ordered thousands of stray cats killed. This didn't help either.

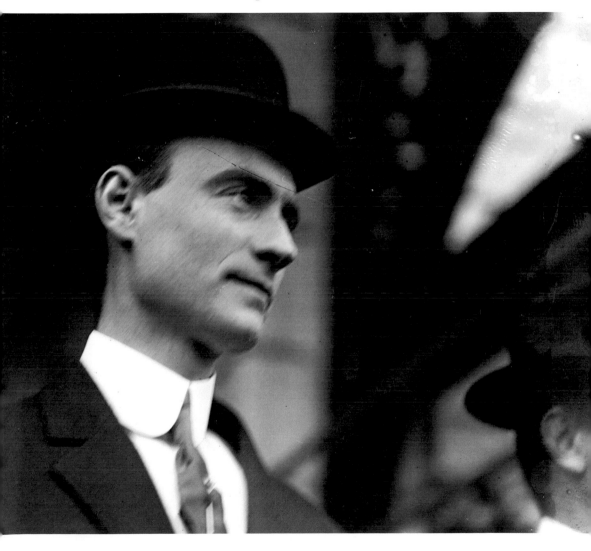

New York City mayor John P. Mitchell was in a tough position. He was expected to protect his city's residents, but no one knew how. Although he did his best, most of his policies and actions accomplished nothing—or made things worse.

Life Under Quarantine

Finally, on July 14, 1916, Mitchell declared a quarantine of the city. No one was allowed to travel outside the city or even to the other boroughs. Children under the age of sixteen were not allowed to go anywhere unless they carried a clean health certificate from their family doctors. Public health notices were posted on trees, in store windows, and at train stations.

New York City changed dramatically as the weeks went by. Movie theaters closed. No one could be found on playgrounds or in libraries. City pools were shut down. No one went to birthday parties, and schoolrooms sat silent and empty.

Let's Play Candy Land

Do you remember those trips through the Peppermint Forest and the Gumdrop Pass? How about finding the Kandy King and outrunning Lord Licorice or stopping by to say hello to Gloppy the Molasses Monster? If these names sound familiar, it is because they were part of the original Candy Land game, invented in the 1940s by a young woman named Eleanor Abbott.

The story behind how she came to invent one of the best-selling children's games of all time is an interesting one. Eleanor Abbott was one of the many young people who suffered from polio. While she was recovering in a San Diego, California, hospital room, she came up with the idea for a simple game that would keep the smallest patients entertained. That idea developed into Candy Land. More than six decades later, it remains one of the top-selling board games for kids.

Neighborhood ball games disappeared. Beaches were deserted, and county fairs were cancelled. Summer camps closed. Restaurants and businesses were shuttered. Even community churches closed their doors.

Families with sick children were desperate, living in great fear and worry. The mayor had given them two choices: They could set up a sanitary room in their homes to care for their children, or they could take their children to the hospital. Although the hospital might sound like the best choice, it wasn't necessarily. With so many young children falling ill, hospitals were overwhelmed. Emergency wards were packed with beds of sick and even dying patients. Doctors and nurses were overworked and exhausted. The hospital was considered a last resort for many.

Before the 1916 epidemic came to an end, it had spread far beyond New York City. By the end of November of that year, twenty-seven thousand people were diagnosed with polio throughout the country. Only a third of these cases were in New York. Of those numbers, 7,000 died in the United States, 2,400 of them New Yorkers. Polio had become the most dreaded disease in the country. Yet it was still a mystery that countless experts were scrambling to understand. Isolation and quarantine—the only two weapons available to doctors and government health officials—were proving to be completely ineffective.

Even the Most Powerful Are Vulnerable

The 1916 polio epidemic brought the disease to the nation's attention. One of its victims, however, cemented the impact of the illness upon American history forever.

It was the summer of 1921. The wealthy and politically connected Roosevelt family was on vacation at Campobello Island, a small place off the coast of the Canadian province of New Brunswick. Franklin D. Roosevelt, future governor of New York and president of the United States, was then working as a lawyer after a failed vice presidential run the year before.

That summer, he, his wife, Eleanor, and their five children were enjoying time at the ocean when Franklin began to feel chilled. The muscles of his right knee and then his left one

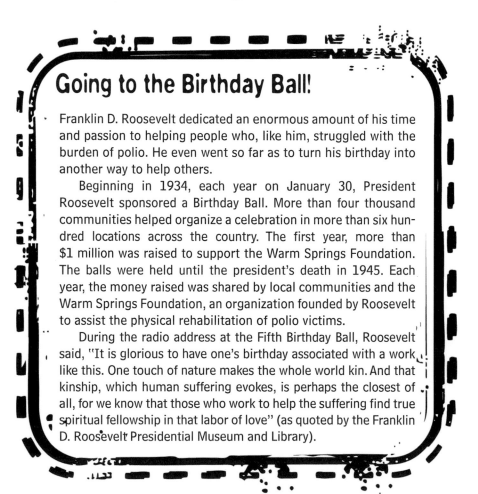

Going to the Birthday Ball!

· Franklin D. Roosevelt dedicated an enormous amount of his time and passion to helping people who, like him, struggled with the burden of polio. He even went so far as to turn his birthday into another way to help others.

Beginning in 1934, each year on January 30, President Roosevelt sponsored a Birthday Ball. More than four thousand communities helped organize a celebration in more than six hundred locations across the country. The first year, more than $1 million was raised to support the Warm Springs Foundation. The balls were held until the president's death in 1945. Each year, the money raised was shared by local communities and the Warm Springs Foundation, an organization founded by Roosevelt to assist the physical rehabilitation of polio victims.

During the radio address at the Fifth Birthday Ball, Roosevelt said, "It is glorious to have one's birthday associated with a work like this. One touch of nature makes the whole world kin. And that kinship, which human suffering evokes, is perhaps the closest of all, for we know that those who work to help the suffering find true spiritual fellowship in that labor of love" (as quoted by the Franklin D. Roosevelt Presidential Museum and Library).

began malfunctioning. Two days later, all the muscles from his chest down were no longer working. Roosevelt eventually regained some strength in his chest but remained paralyzed from the waist down for the rest of his life.

Although doctors first suspected a blood clot on the spine, they finally determined it was polio (though some modern researchers believe Roosevelt may actually have had Guillain-Barré syndrome, an autoimmune disorder that affects the central nervous system). For an adult man to contract what was typically considered a children's disease was shocking. That this man was so prominent in social, financial, and political circles made it even more so.

A Politician Struggles to Protect the Public While Hiding His Condition

Franklin D. Roosevelt worked hard to conceal the extent of his illness. Thousands of photos exist of him, yet only two depict him in a wheelchair. Roosevelt was afraid that his paralysis would ruin his political career by making him appear weak and vulnerable to the American people. So he used leg braces and leaned on podiums and other people's arms for support. He put himself through a series of agonizing exercises to develop his upper body strength. He pulled himself up flights of stairs and dragged himself across the room using only his arms. His bravery in the face of such a disease—and his years of passionate support for finding a cure and helping other victims—helped him become one of the most beloved presidents of all time. After being elected in 1933, he was reelected three more times (he died three months into his fourth term).

Despite Roosevelt's best efforts, the poliovirus kept attacking the public, still targeting its youngest members. In

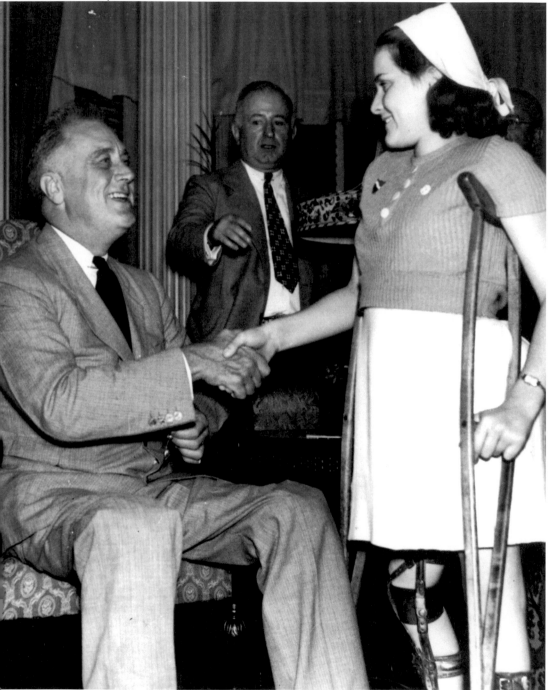

Franklin D. Roosevelt made it a special point to meet and talk with many young polio victims. He made the disease a high priority throughout his four presidential terms.

1934, Los Angeles, California, saw more than 2,500 cases of polio. More cases followed across the country throughout the 1930s and 1940s. After World War II ended, the nation experienced more than twenty thousand cases from 1945 to 1949. Neighbors discussed the latest outbreaks in hushed and anxious tones. Children lived under a dark cloud of fear. Magazine articles discussed the disease. Reporters analyzed the latest medical efforts. Scientists searched for breakthroughs. Physicians tried new treatments. Charitable research organizations like the March of Dimes were formed, and the donations poured in. The fight was on—but the biggest polio epidemic was still ahead.

CHAPTER THREE

FAMILIES SUFFER AND SOCIETY MARCHES TO WAR AGAINST POLIO

As much damage as polio could do to people's bodies, it did just as much harm to their families. Summertime—a time of freedom, sunshine, fun, and celebration—turned into a time of dread and fear. Children were closely guarded by terrified parents and kept indoors and away from crowds. Polio was a disease that no one seemed to be able to predict or understand. It was an invisible enemy that knew how to destroy the most vulnerable of victims: children. The slightest sniffle or the smallest ache was cause for panic. Parents knew that a diagnosis of polio meant many things:

- Financial stress (medicine and equipment were expensive)
- Pain and suffering (treatments were often extremely uncomfortable, especially for little ones)
- Isolation (families were quarantined and isolated from the rest of the community)
- Social stigma (people who were infected were often shunned)
- And, worst of all, permanent paralysis or even death

26

Wilma Rudolph

When Wilma Rudolph was born prematurely in 1940 in Clarksville, Tennessee, it seemed unlikely that, one day, she would inspire countless children and athletes to do their best.

From the beginning, Rudolph was not a healthy child. She spent weeks in bed with pneumonia and scarlet fever. Then, when she was only four years old, she was diagnosed with polio. She lost the use of her left leg, and doctors told her parents that she would never walk again.

At six, she was given metal leg braces. "I spent most of my time trying to figure out how to get them off," she later admitted (as quoted by ESPN). As the twentieth of twenty-two children in her family, she had lots of brothers and sisters who offered to massage her leg. Once a week, her mother drove her 90 miles (145 kilometers) roundtrip to a hospital for therapy with Sister Kenny. It took years of treatment, but by age nine, Rudolph's braces were off. At age eleven, she discovered basketball. From that point on, her life revolved around sports.

Yet it was only when she discovered track that she truly blossomed athletically. She ran so fast that she earned nicknames like the "Black Gazelle." She ran for the U.S. Olympic team in 1956 and won the bronze in the 400-meter relay. Four years later, she returned and took home three gold medals. Later, she worked as a coach and served as a U.S. Goodwill Ambassador to French West Africa. Her advice to other athletes was a reminder that "triumph can't be had without the struggle" (as quoted by ESPN).

Struggling Children, Exhausted Mothers, Isolated Families

For children, being diagnosed with polio meant life would never be quite the same again. Not only did they have to deal with not feeling well but also with not being able to play with their friends or go to school. It frequently meant being separated from their families as they were put in isolated hospital

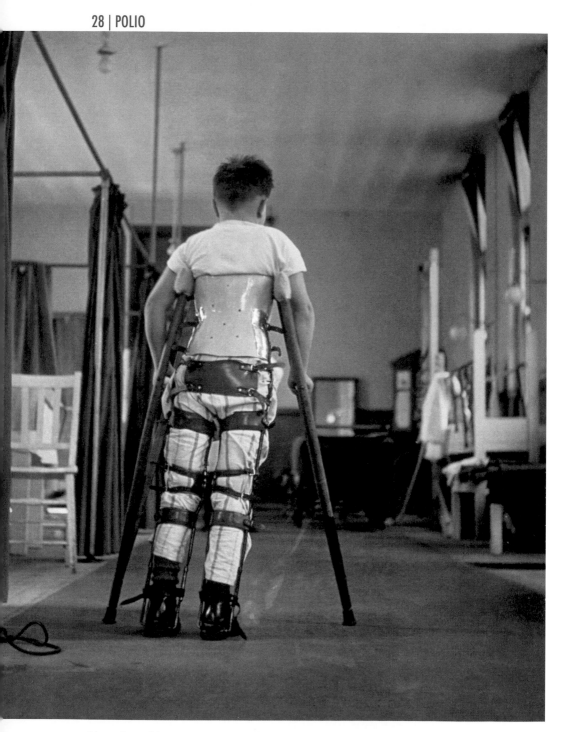

Heartbreaking images like this one were sometimes used to remind people to get the polio vaccine once it was available and encourage them to send in donations to fight against the disease.

rooms and only allowed to communicate through masks and glass windows.

When these children finally got to come back home, life did not always go back to normal. First, they had to deal with whatever lingering effects polio had left them with—from ongoing fatigue to a slight limp to paralysis. They might have to adapt to 10 pounds (4.5 kg) of metal leg braces or prepare for upcoming surgery. Often their bedrooms had been transformed into hospital-like rooms, and their belongings and clothing were destroyed for fear that any of it still harbored the poliovirus. A simple trip to the bathroom became challenging or even impossible.

Mothers often had to deal with enormous responsibilities during these times. They had to wear multiple hats, from nurse to mother to teacher. They spent their days attending to the needs of their sick children—doing everything from doling out medicine to carrying heat packs, changing sheets, and emptying and cleaning bedpans. They comforted with hugs, entertained with stories, educated with schoolbooks, and did all they could to make this terrible time a little bit easier. It was a huge role to play and an exhausting one.

In 1952, one of the biggest polio epidemics of all hit the country. Victims numbered almost fifty-eight thousand, and deaths rose to more than three thousand. Hundreds of victims were paralyzed. It was one of the darkest moments in American history and one that had everyone crying out for a solution. This time, mercifully, a solution was not far away.

The American Public Joins the March of Dimes

Polio victims and their families desperately needed help and support, and President Roosevelt recognized this growing need. He asked Basil O'Connor, his friend and business manager, to help him. In 1938, the two men created the National Foundation for Infantile Paralysis.

The organization was a combination of volunteers who wanted to help and educate victims and scientists who were given funds to do further research. It was promoted by some of the biggest Hollywood stars of the time, including Judy Garland and Mickey Rooney. This national fund-raiser asked people to give whatever they possibly could to help bring an end to polio. Instead of turning to the few millionaires for large donations, it pursued the idea, for the first time, of looking to millions of ordinary people for tiny donations.

The well-known comedian and actor Eddie Cantor accidentally helped coin the nickname for the organization when

The Man Behind the March

The name Eddie Cantor (1892–1964) is not a familiar one to today's younger generation. But to American audiences of the early twentieth century, he was one of the most famous personalities on the planet. He was a singer, actor, and comedian who appeared on radio and television and was known as "Banjo Eyes" because of his large, expressive eyes.

Along with his talent as an entertainer, Cantor was also a humanitarian. He enthusiastically jumped in to help promote President Roosevelt's National Foundation for Infantile Paralysis. He helped organize the first radio campaign, enlisting the help of some other popular entertainers of the day such as Bing Crosby, Jack Benny, and ventriloquist Edgar Bergen and his dummy Charlie McCarthy. It was a tremendous success that helped the March of Dimes become a powerful organization.

In 1962, Israel gave Cantor the Medallion of Valor for his many humanitarian efforts. He died in 1964 at the age of seventy-two.

he asked everyone to contribute anything they could—even something as small as a dime. He promoted the idea on radio shows, calling for a "March of Dimes."

The name stuck. President Roosevelt stated, "In sending a dime . . . and in dancing that others may walk, we the people are striking a powerful blow in defense of American freedom and human decency" (as quoted by the FDR Presidential Library and Museum). Cantor added, "The March of Dimes will enable all persons, even the children, to show our President that they are with him in this battle against this disease. Nearly everyone can send in a dime, or several dimes," he added. "However, it only takes ten dimes to make a dollar, and if a million people send only one dime, the total will be $100,000" (as quoted by the March of Dimes).

A dime does not seem like a very helpful donation by today's standards, but it is important to realize that in the 1930s and 1940s, a dime could buy a quart of milk, a hot dog, subway fare, or a hot cup of coffee. At first, the response to this call for a dime donation met with little response. In fact, only $17.50 had been sent in two days later. Had the appeal failed? No, it had just taken a while to reach Americans across the nation.

Within three weeks, more than eighty thousand letters containing dimes—and more—flooded the mailroom at the White House. In all, more than $268,000 was donated. Roosevelt was stunned. He went on the radio and said, "During the past few days, bags of mail have been coming, literally by the truck-load, to the White House . . . how many I cannot tell you, for we can only estimate the actual count by counting the mailbags. In all the envelopes are dimes and quarters and even dollar bills—gifts from grown-ups and children—mostly from children who want to help other children to get well" (as quoted by the March of Dimes).

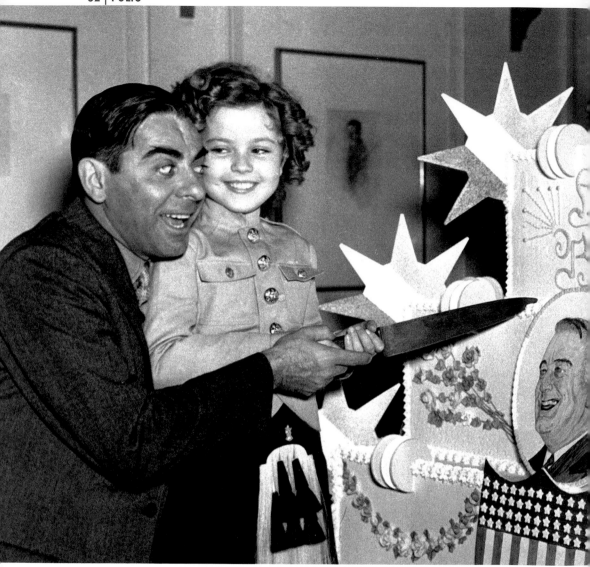

In 1937, comedian Eddie Cantor and child film star Shirley Temple help celebrate President Franklin Roosevelt's birthday in Los Angeles, California.

A Society Awakened, Motivated, and Mobilized

Although fund-raisers like the March of Dimes are common today, at the time this one was organized, it was the first of

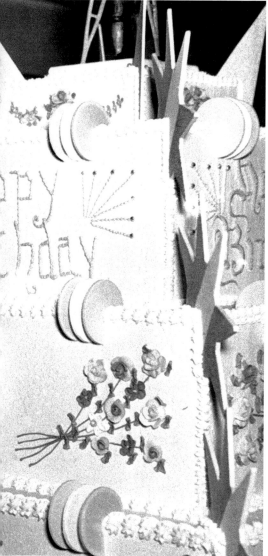

its kind. No other organization had ever turned to everyday citizens and asked for their help in finding an answer to a threat of disease.

March of Dimes posters featuring illustrations of children in leg braces and wheelchairs were put up everywhere. Donation canisters were put outside the doors of stores and businesses. People went door-to-door asking for contributions. Dozens of different kinds of events were held to raise money for the organization, including square dances, stock car races, radio marathons, and school talent shows. The money each of these events generated was used for training medical professionals in how to take care of polio patients. The funds also helped patients with the cost of therapy, treatment, medicine, and equipment.

When donations began to falter, O'Connor tried a different tactic: fear. He created a media campaign that reminded the American people that polio can strike anyone, anywhere, at any time, so they should keep those donations coming in. Short films portraying polio as a dark and menacing shadow that stalked young children were shown before movie features—a reminder that the threat was ever present. The people responded, and soon the organization was receiving an astonishing $22 million a year in donations.

Today, the March of Dimes no longer targets polio, as it has been nearly eradicated (eliminated) throughout the world.

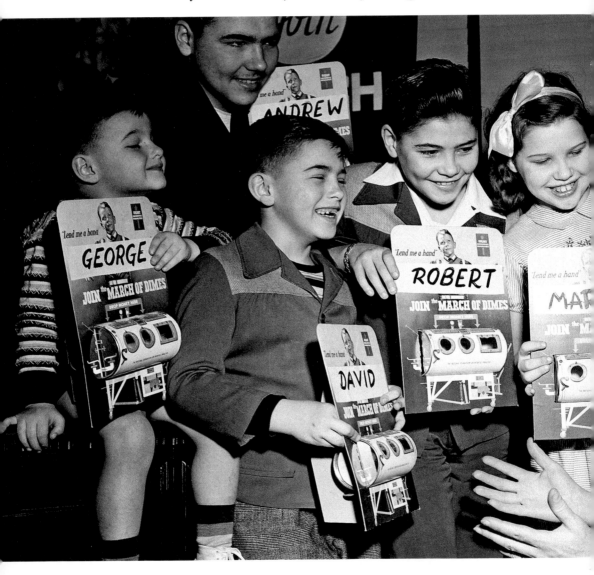

All five children in the Schofield family of Newark, New Jersey, were struck with polio and hospitalized. It was the greatest incidence of polio among siblings reported. The brothers and sisters are seen here turning over the money they raised for the March of Dimes to Basil O'Connor in 1955.

Instead, its new focus is on birth defects and putting a stop to them through an ongoing March of Dimes.

Thanks to the wildly successful fund-raising efforts of the March of Dimes, help was on the way to polio victims, but

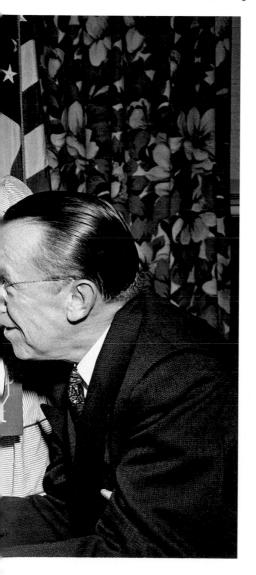

answers were still eluding the best scientific researchers. In the meantime, the medical world was struggling to adapt to the complications of coping with sporadic epidemics. Even as the race for a cure got underway, most doctors were simply trying to find a way to treat polio's debilitating symptoms and care for the disease's deeply suffering victims.

CHAPTER FOUR

THE MEDICAL ESTABLISHMENT STRUGGLES TO FIND SOLUTIONS

As researchers conducted experiment after experiment in the hopes of finding a successful polio vaccine, doctors were scrambling to find the best way to treat the youngest victims of polio. In the nineteenth century, methods were crude, painful, and typically unsuccessful. Bleeding—a cure-all for many medical conditions—was frequently used. Doctors also sometimes applied ice to the spines of patients, followed by an ointment made of mercury to create blisters. Electrical currents were sent through paralyzed limbs in the hope of "waking" them up. Some doctors felt applying a red-hot iron to the afflicted body part was a good idea, while others thought amputation was the best choice.

By the twentieth century, doctors had new theories, most of them far-fetched. One idea was that polio patients would be cured if they went horseback riding. Another was that they needed to be exposed to ultraviolet (UV) light. Some doctors had patients soak in saltwater baths.

Water Therapy

The idea of soaking in water was one that intrigued President Roosevelt. In 1924, he decided that soaking in natural hot springs might make his muscles work better, so he traveled to the Warm

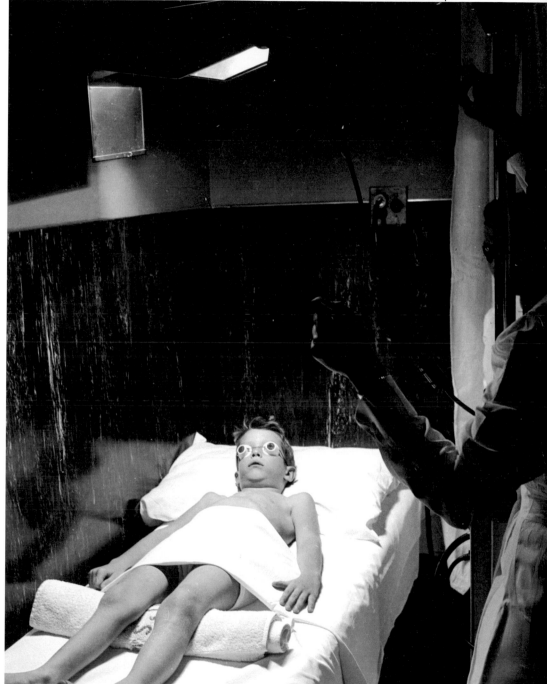

In some hospitals, young polio sufferers were put under UV light to see if that would help treat the disease and its symptoms. Protective glasses were worn to shield the eyes.

Springs resort in Georgia. He found that the water did relax him and allow him to move in ways he could not on land.

Roosevelt began making regular visits to the springs. Eventually, he decided not only to build a home there, known

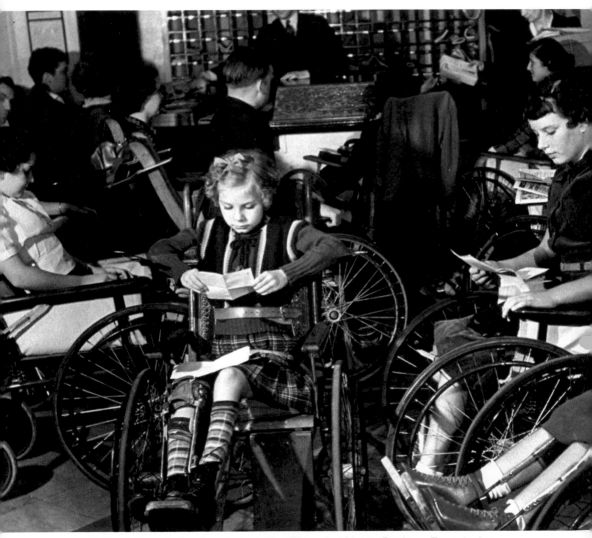

Polio victims being treated at the Georgia Warm Springs Foundation kept in touch with their families through letters. In between treatments, they gathered around the mail room desk and eagerly read of home-town happenings.

as the Little White House, but also to buy the entire property and turn it into a rehabilitation center for other polio patients to use. He named it the Roosevelt Warm Springs Institute for Rehabilitation. Between 1924 and his death in 1945, the president made more than forty trips to soak in the hot springs.

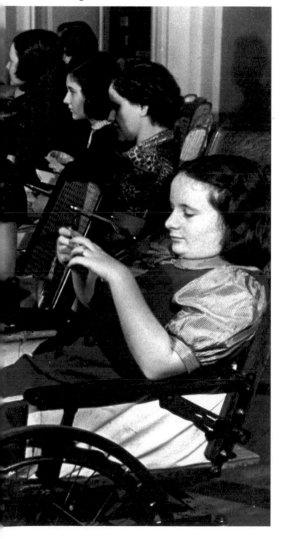

They did not prove to be a cure, but they were soothing. The president was at Warm Springs when he passed away in 1945 of a massive stroke.

Immobilization

Although soaking in hot water did help some patients' muscles feel better, the prevailing medical thought was that the best way to treat polio patients was to immobilize them (keep them from moving). Doctors hoped this would lessen the pain and help the muscles to heal. In order to keep patients still, they put wooden splints and plaster casts on children's arms and legs. Some patients endured body wedging, in which the body was wrapped in a knee-to-armpit cast and a block of wood was inserted in the cast to force the spine straight. Over time, larger and larger pieces of wood were used.

Many of the children were strapped down in hospital beds that were equipped with ropes and pulleys to keep them completely still. Although the intentions of the doctors were honorable, this was a horrible way to live day after day, week after week, especially for young children. It did enormous damage to their developing skeletons. Encased in casts and unable to move, the muscles became atrophied, or weakened. Legs did not grow at the same rate. And once the casts and splints were removed, children frequently needed leg braces, crutches, canes, orthopedic shoes, or wheelchairs. A number of surgeries to realign short legs, fuse joints, lengthen tendons, or straighten spines were required to correct the damage that polio—and its well-intentioned treatments—inflicted.

Life Inside the Iron Lung

Doctors used casts and splints to deal with polio-stricken arms and legs, but what could they do to help the patients whose chest muscles were too paralyzed to allow them to breathe easily? Many of these people died slow and painful deaths, literally suffocating due to their inability to draw breath.

All of that changed in 1927 with the invention of the respirator, a breathing machine invented by engineers Philip Drinker and Louis Agassiz Shaw from Harvard University. It was designed to help keep people breathing until they were able to do so on their own. The machine was made out of a cylindrical metal tank and powered by an electric motor with two vacuum cleaners. The pump altered the atmospheric pressure inside the tank, allowing air to be pulled in and out of the patient's lungs. It was called a respirator but was quickly given the nickname "iron lung." Patients who were forced to

Inside Tuskegee

Although the poliovirus did not discriminate when it chose its victims, the hospitals and medical centers that took care of polio patients often did. It was a time of segregation in many parts of the country, years before the civil rights movement achieved progress for African Americans. The Roosevelt Warm Springs Institute for Rehabilitation, founded in 1927 by Franklin D. Roosevelt in Warm Springs, Georgia, opened its doors to the poor—but not to African Americans. Where could they go when polio struck? Many of them went to Tuskegee, Alabama, to the John A. Andrew Memorial Hospital. It opened a polio center in 1941, funded by the March of Dimes.

The Tuskegee Institute had been established by Dr. George Washington Carver, known for his experimentation with peanuts and their products, including peanut butter, peanut diesel fuel, and peanut oil. Carver used the peanut oil to massage the legs of polio patients. The school also offered courses on orthopedic shoe and leg brace construction.

spend time inside one had to learn to let the machine do the breathing for them—not an easy thing to do.

The sight of a small child encased in one of these tubes, with nothing but his or her head sticking out, was a heart-breaking one. Round portholes lined the sides of the tube, allowing medical personnel to reach in and adjust the patient's arms and legs, change the bed sheets, or apply heat packs. Creative parents and medical workers helped make the time a little easier to bear by inventing ways to hold books above the children's faces or beam movies on the ceiling overhead. Mirrors were positioned over the heads of patients so they could see the faces of visitors and doctors when they stopped by. Still, most memoirs written by children who were required

Finding a way to pass the hours while in an iron lung was crucial, especially for children. Reading comic books and other materials held overhead was one possible entertaining distraction from pain, boredom, and loneliness.

to stay inside these machines speak of long, lonely hours and feelings of isolation and depression.

As helpful as the iron lungs were, they were also costly and cumbersome, taking up as much room on a hospital floor as a small car. Each one cost approximately $1,500—the same

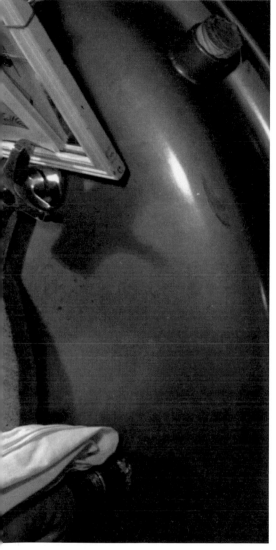

price as the average home of that time period. Most families could not afford to have one in their homes. Instead, they relied on the hospitals' supply of the equipment, which was not always extensive. The available supply did not always meet the demands of the swelling number of polio patients. This also meant that afflicted children who were lucky enough to gain access to a hospital's iron lung were away from home for weeks or even months, lying in a lonely hospital ward and separated from their families. Despite the cost and inconvenience of the machines, the manufacturers of the iron lungs could barely keep up with the demand.

In 1931, inventor John Haven Emerson created a new and improved version of the machine that cost less. Soon hospitals were equipped with rows of the cylinders filled with patients who remained there until they could again breathe on their own, usually one to two weeks. Although the iron lungs never cured anyone of polio, they saved many lives by providing patients with paralyzed chest muscles the ability to breathe until their bodies could again perform that job on their own.

The Kenny Method

When Elizabeth Kenny (1886–1952) was a teenager grow-ing up in Australia, she broke her wrist. Little did she know that this simple injury would not only determine her life's profession but would also change the lives of countless young polio victims.

As the doctor treated her injured wrist, Kenny became fascinated by the world of medicine. As a result, she trained as a nurse at a private hospital in Sydney. She then spent time in the Australian outback taking care of the indigenous tribes who lived there. During World War I, she worked as a nurse in the army, acquiring the nickname Sister Kenny

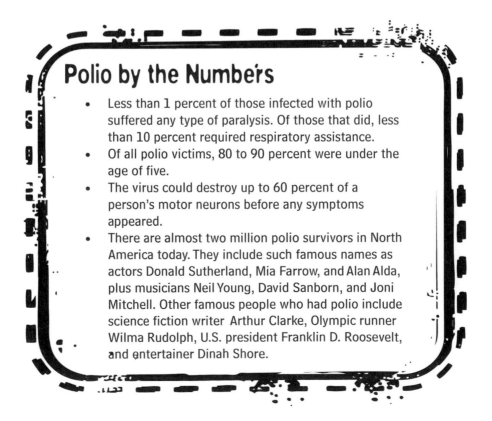

Polio by the Numbers

- Less than 1 percent of those infected with polio suffered any type of paralysis. Of those that did, less than 10 percent required respiratory assistance.
- Of all polio victims, 80 to 90 percent were under the age of five.
- The virus could destroy up to 60 percent of a person's motor neurons before any symptoms appeared.
- There are almost two million polio survivors in North America today. They include such famous names as actors Donald Sutherland, Mia Farrow, and Alan Alda, plus musicians Neil Young, David Sanborn, and Joni Mitchell. Other famous people who had polio include science fiction writer Arthur Clarke, Olympic runner Wilma Rudolph, U.S. president Franklin D. Roosevelt, and entertainer Dinah Shore.

(experienced nurses in England and Australia are referred to as "Sister").

When a polio epidemic hit Queensland in 1933, Kenny opened a number of clinics throughout Australia. Her ideas on how to treat the disease, however, were in direct opposition to medical thought at the time. It took years for the so-called Kenny method to be accepted in her homeland, and even longer to be adopted as common practice in the United States.

Sister Kenny believed that keeping a patient's muscles immobilized was a terrible mistake. In her experience, a muscle that spasms, or contracts involuntarily, needs to be massaged and exercised in order to relax, increase the blood flow, and heal properly. Her recommended treatment for polio victims was the application of hot, wet packs or blankets to the afflicted areas, followed by stretching of the muscles. It was a painful type of treatment. Children often cried when their muscles, after weeks of being kept immobile, were moved and stretched. However, as time passed, these children also frequently improved greatly. They also healed better and became more mobile than those children receiving standard immobilizing treatments.

It took some time for the American medical establishment to accept Sister Kenny's methods. The ideas were quite radical to doctors who had been taught to bind muscles and prevent movement. Finally, Basil O'Connor, head of the National Foundation for Infantile Paralysis, officially stated, "The length of time during which pain, tenderness, and spasm are present is greatly reduced and contractures caused by muscle shortening during . . . [the early] period are prevented by the Kenny method. The general physical condition of the patients receiving this treatment seems to

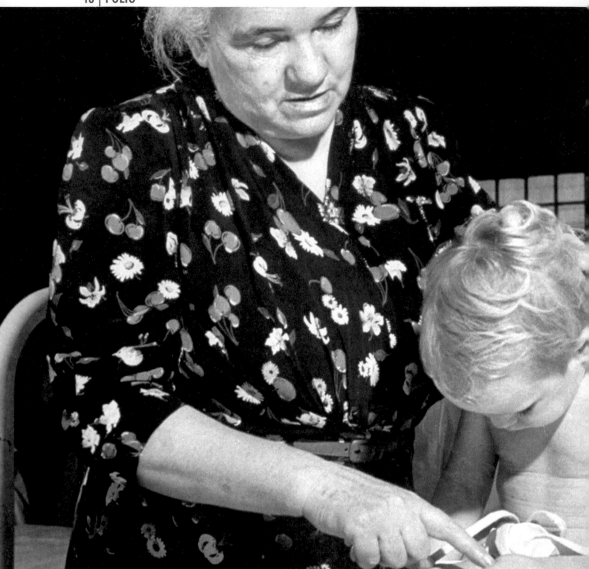

During her presentations to American nurses and physicians, Sister Kenny often used young patients to demonstrate her innovative and, for the time, radical methods for treating muscles ravaged by polio.

be better than that of patients treated by some of the other methods" (as quoted by *Time* magazine).

In December 1942, Kenny opened the Sister Elizabeth Kenny Institute in Minneapolis and began training other

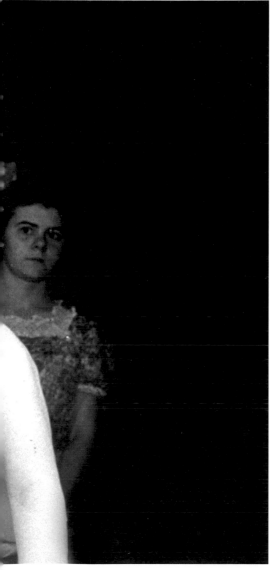

medical professionals to use her methods. For her revolutionary work, she was given numerous awards and honors. In 1946, a movie was made about Sister Kenny's life, starring the actress Rosalind Russell.

Sister Kenny died in 1952, at the age of seventy-two, three years before the discovery of a successful polio vaccine. Though she didn't live to see this happy day, her own methods of treatment and rehabilitation for polio victims had finally gained worldwide acceptance by the end of her lifetime. She had the satisfaction of knowing that her work was helping save the lives and limbs of polio's young victims.

CHAPTER FIVE

THE RACE TO DEVELOP A VACCINE

With the passing of each summer, the desperation for a way to prevent or to cure infection with poliovirus grew. As America's worst epidemic swept across the country, Basil O'Connor made a dramatic announcement in 1953: He had a vaccine that was ready to be tested on the nation's children. People everywhere rejoiced, but a few had their doubts about whether this was the wisest move.

O'Connor had been pushing hard for a vaccine for years. In his position with the March of Dimes, he felt the growing pressure for a solution and it was exhausting. Where was the medical researcher who would have just the right combination of skills, knowledge, and practical experience to draw upon to create a successful vaccine?

Early Promise and Disappointing Failures

Numerous scientists had been working on the problem, of course, but progress was slow. Two people seemed to be at the head of the race: Maurice Brodie and John Kollmer. Both were so

With Rights for All

Not all of polio's effects on the nation were harmful. The disease had an enormous impact on disability rights in the United States. In 1935, the League of the Physically Handicapped was established in New York. Many of the founders were polio survivors who had encountered job discrimination because of their disabilities.

As the epidemics of the 1950s grew, the sight of people walking on crutches, wearing leg braces, or using a wheelchair became very familiar. Their presence helped remind people that disabilities were not just a medical issue, but social and civil rights issues as well. The large numbers of disabled polio survivors brought attention to the need to make public places accessible. That meant that modifications to public buildings and spaces needed to be made, such as wheelchair ramps, electric doors, and elevators.

In 1968, the Architectural Barriers Act was passed. It stated that all buildings that were designed, built, or leased with federal money must be equipped with ramps, curb cuts, and open access to everyone. In 1990, polio survivors were highly instrumental in getting the equally groundbreaking Americans with Disabilities Act passed. This act fuather protected disabled citizens from discrimination and ensured their access to all aspects of public life. Something good had come out of the polio scourge.

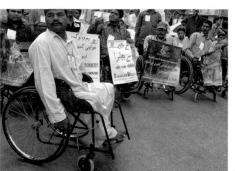

Pakistani polio victims stage a demonstration against the government's health officials who had temporarily withheld polio vaccinations.

determined to be the first to invent a polio vaccine that they rushed the process. In 1935, Brodie tested his vaccine on three thousand children. It was made from the ground-up spinal cords of infected monkeys. The virus had been deactivated by a mixture of formaldehyde and other chemicals. No one is sure what happened next. History books simply state that something went wrong. Whatever that "something" was, it was serious, and all trials were suddenly discontinued.

Kollmer came at it from a different angle. He believed the vaccine should have a live, but weakened, virus. Like Brodie, he used the virus from infected monkeys, mixed it with chemicals, and then put it in the refrigerator for two weeks. He injected it into himself, his family, and two dozen other volunteers. When there seemed to be no ill effects, he sent thousands of doses to physicians. Sadly, his vaccine did not work and, in fact, caused polio in some people. Speaking at the American Public Health Association later, as quoted by Edmund Sass in *Polio's Legacy: An Oral History*, he stated, "Gentlemen, this is one time I wish the floor would open up and swallow me."

Polio Pioneers: Jonas Salk and the First Vaccinated Children

The day when Basil O'Connor first met Jonas Salk, a professor of bacteriology at the University of Pittsburgh, was an important one. Both men were driven to succeed in life and were passionate about ending polio. O'Connor was positive he had finally found the man who would lead the country out of fear and ill health. He did all he could to encourage and support Salk's research. He was so confident that Salk would find the answer to polio that he made his famous announcement that a vaccine was just around the corner.

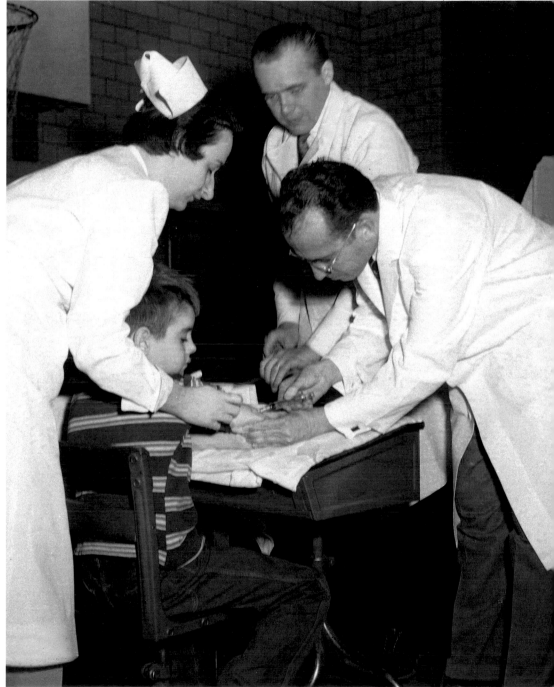

The public was so eager for a cure for polio that children were vaccinated sitting at their school desks. Dr. Salk administers the shot to a small boy in Pittsburgh, Pennsylvania, in 1954.

Now, the pressure was on in the Salk lab. The world had been alerted to an imminent polio vaccine and was anxiously watching and waiting. It took months for O'Connor's promise of a safe and effective vaccine to be realized. Vaccine trials were performed secretly at the D. T. Watson Home for Crippled Children outside Pittsburgh, Pennsylvania. Salk even administered the experimental vaccine to himself and his family members. Following these tests, Salk concluded that the time had come to announce a breakthrough.

In November 1953, O'Connor told the American public that a vaccine was ready to be tested on the nation's children. It was one of the most massive science experiments in the history of the country. The vaccine, composed of the dead and deactivated virus, had relatively little testing done and had gone through only small trials. Compared to the stringent standards and regulations in place today, administering the unproven vaccine to the nation's children was a huge risk.

The fear of polio was greater than the fear of the vaccine, however, and within six months, more than two million children, proudly nicknamed the "Polio Pioneers," had been vaccinated. Then the world held its breath and waited for summer to return. Would the vaccine be effective? Would children's bodies have developed the antibodies they needed to provide lifelong immunity to this invisible enemy?

On March 12, 1955, every other news story took a backseat to an announcement from the March of Dimes. Reporters lined up, cameras flashed, and typewriters stood ready as the verdict was given: Salk's polio vaccine appeared to be a complete success. It was safe, potent, and effective. Factory whistles blew, children cheered, car horns honked, and parents wept with relief. Newspaper headlines were the same all over the country: The Salk Vaccine Is a Success!

A Tragic Setback

This explosive burst of joy and relief was short-lived, however. A month later, the surgeon general came on television to announce that the polio vaccine program was being halted temporarily. More than two hundred of those children immunized had gotten polio anyway. More than 150 of these victims were now paralyzed. A handful had even died.

An investigation quickly determined that all of those children who developed severe illness had received the vaccine from a shipment made by Cutter Laboratories in California. The company had accidentally released a contaminated batch of vaccine that still contained the live poliovirus. This accident helped lead to the many rules and regulations that are in place today for scientific laboratories.

Having discovered the source of the problem and fixed it, the vaccination program was restarted only eight days after it had been halted. There was no question now that the Salk vaccine was successful. The number of polio cases began to drop quickly. In the first year of the program, the number of polio cases decreased from 35,000 to 5,600. When the Sabin vaccine replaced the Salk vaccine in 1962, the rate of effectiveness increased even further. In 1964, there were only 121 cases reported throughout the United States.

The numbers dropped every year after that, and, by 1994, polio had been completely eradicated in the United States. Children born today are given a series of polio vaccinations at two months, four months, and between six to eighteen months of age. A booster shot is also given between the ages of four and six.

Thanks to the hard work, dedication, determination, and courage of millions of people—the youthful Polio Pioneers most especially—across the nation, a medical nightmare that had haunted humanity for hundreds, even thousands, of years had finally come to an end. The poliovirus's silent army was defeated at long last.

A Dissenting Voice

While the world's eyes were on Jonas Salk, another researcher was also hard at work trying to create a safe and effective polio vaccine. His name was Dr. Albert Sabin, a pediatrician from Poland who had come to the United States in 1921. During World War II, he served in the Army Medical Corps, working on vaccines for hepatitis, dengue fever, and Japanese encephalitis.

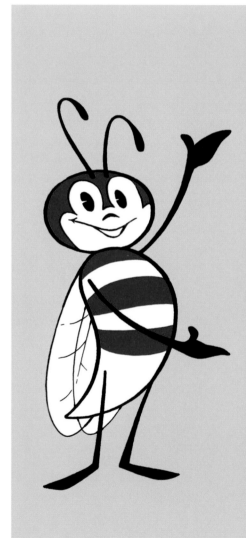

Sabin's years of lab and research experience convinced him that Salk's vaccine was not as effective as it should be. While Salk used a dead, deactivated virus that was injected into the bloodstream, Sabin's vaccine used a live virus that was taken orally (via the mouth) in drops. Sabin was very worried that Salk was hurrying his vaccine and that this rush would result in tragedy. He spoke out about it often, but his voice went largely unheard. The public was so desperate for some good news on the polio front that someone expressing doubt, skepticism, and a desire to slow down the vaccination development process was not given a fair hearing. In any case, his voice of caution was drowned out by the forceful,

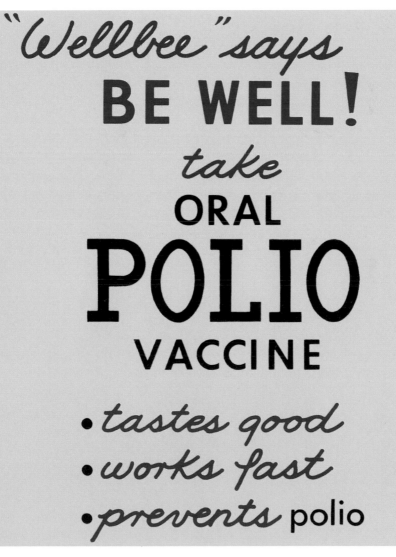

The image of the "Wellbee" was a familiar one to schoolchildren in the 1960s. His image, created by the Centers for Disease Control and Prevention, appeared on posters, newspapers, fliers, and television commercials. Wellbee became the national symbol of public health.

influential, and optimistic pronouncements of Salk, O'Connor, and the March of Dimes.

When the bad batch of Salk vaccines from Cutter Laboratories was discovered, Sabin's warnings proved to be valid. When his own vaccine was ready for mass use in 1955, however, he was overlooked once more. So Sabin took his vaccine to other countries where it was used very successfully. In 1960, Sabin's vaccine was finally licensed for use in the United States. By 1965, it was the primary one used because it was cheaper to make and easier to administer.

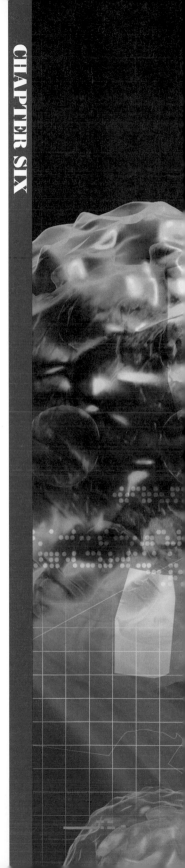

CHAPTER SIX

POLIO TODAY

For younger generations of Americans, polio is primarily something that is learned about in health or history classes. It is only the second disease for which eradication by science has been attempted on a global scale (smallpox was the first and was successful). Eradication of polio from the United States is one of the country's proudest accomplishments. However, polio has not completely disappeared from the planet—or even from the United States. Its presence still lurks in a handful of other nations, and unfortunately, in recent years, it has resurfaced in the United States as well.

The last case of "wild" polio in the United States (caused by the live poliovirus, rather than the vaccination) was in 1979. The rare cases that have appeared since then have been traced to the use of Sabin's oral polio vaccine. Some countries are still dealing with wild polio outbreaks, however, including India, Afghanistan, Nigeria, and Pakistan.

Eradicating Polio Worldwide

Programs like the Global Polio Eradication Initiative (GPEI) are working hard to put an end to

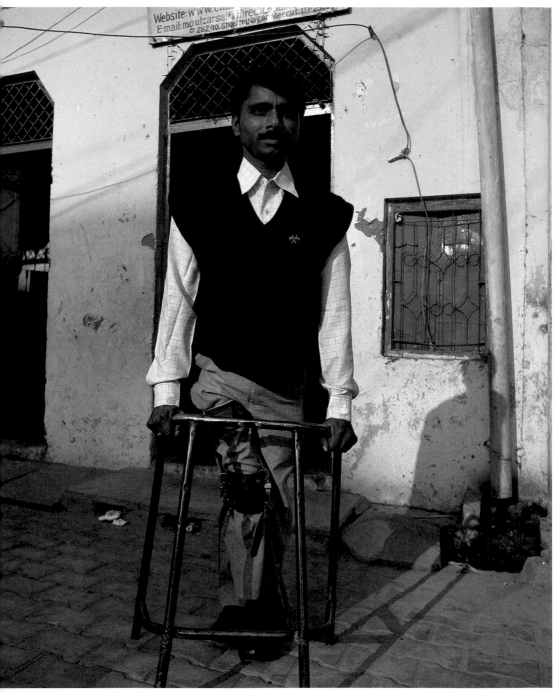

Polio victim Mohammad Bulzar Saifi, a twenty-five-year-old man from northern India, was the focus of an Oscar-nominated documentary called *The Final Inch*, about global efforts to eradicate polio throughout the world.

polio in even the most remote parts of the world. GPEI is a joint venture of several organizations: the World Health Organization (WHO), the Centers for Disease Control and Prevention (CDC), the United Nations Children's Fund (UNICEF), and Rotary International, a service club organization with more than one million members. GPEI was established in 1988 with the goal of eradicating polio worldwide.

These intense, massive vaccination programs are complex but successful events. For example, in January 2001, 150 million children under the age of five were immunized in India. In December 2008, the GPEI coordinated the vaccination of twenty-two million children under the age of five in Bangladesh. This effort took place at over 140,000 sites and involved more than 600,000 volunteers.

When the GPEI started, the poliovirus still existed in more than 125 countries on five different continents. Over the years, GPEI has immunized more than two billion children in two hundred countries. It provides four doses of the oral polio vaccine to children during the first year of life and sponsors National Immunization Days. In addition, GPEI serves as a watchdog, monitoring the emergence of any possible cases of polio. In the event of an outbreak, GPEI sponsors "mop

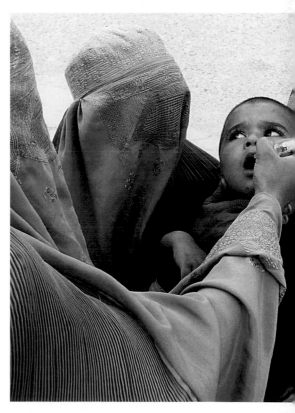

Afghan health workers drop polio vaccine into the mouth of a young child. Afghanistan is one of the only countries left in the world that still has new cases of polio reported each year.

up" campaigns with door-to-door immunizations in high-risk communities.

How is it possible to vaccinate millions of children at the same time? It is not an easy task. Multiple sites have to be organized and thousands of volunteers signed up. The oral vaccine has to be kept at a certain temperature. This, in turn, requires a network of refrigerators and coolers to be hauled through steamy jungles and sandy deserts. They are transported on everything from horses and camels to canoes and motorbikes.

National Immunization Days

In countries that have continued to struggle to eradicate the polio virus, public health organizations have organized National Immunization Days. Volunteers wearing caps, vests, and armbands administer the oral polio vaccine to countless children. The first one was held in Brazil in 1980. A cute character known as the Little Drop (referring to the oral vaccine drops) was featured on banners and signs. This friendly cartoon character was designed to lessen children's fear of vaccination.

What happens if the country where the National Immunization Days are being held is in the middle of a violent civil war? It has happened in the past. Walking through war zones and street battles to get to a hospital or clinic can be terrifying and dangerous, perhaps even deadly. Amazingly enough, whenever war appears to prevent distribution of the polio vaccine, an official "Day of Tranquility" is declared. Both sides put down their weapons, and a temporary cease-fire is declared. All vaccination program volunteers are allowed safe passage, as are the people lined up to get their vaccines. In 1985, for example, in the middle of a civil war in El Salvador,

NATIONAL IMMUNISATION DAYS
1st round: 4th - 5th November, 1998
2nd round: 9th - 10th December, 1998

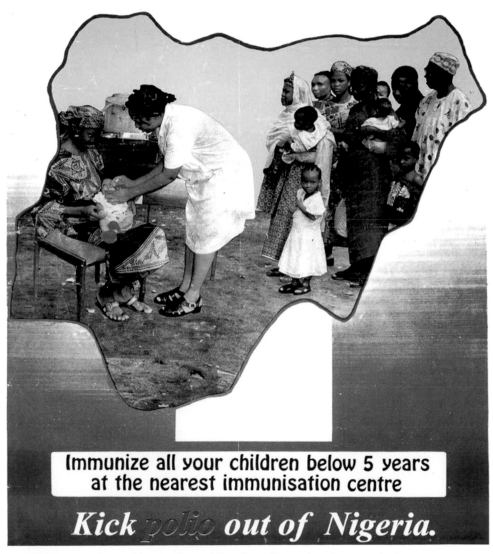

Immunize all your children below 5 years at the nearest immunisation centre

Kick polio out of Nigeria.

Posters, such as this one from Nigeria, tell people where and when to go for polio immunizations. During these special vaccination days, volunteers are able to vaccinate and protect a very large number of children in a very short period of time.

three days of peace were declared so that children could be vaccinated against polio. Similar Days of Tranquility have occurred in Uganda, Lebanon, Sudan, and Sierra Leone.

A Haunting Return?

As if suffering through polio once was not enough, a growing number of polio victims have been reporting a return of symptoms as they age. Statistics vary, but between 25 and 60 percent of those who were sick with polio in childhood have found themselves suffering from a slowly developing set of symptoms that seem hauntingly familiar:

- Exhaustion
- Progressive muscle and joint pain and weakness
- Muscle atrophy
- Breathing or swallowing problems
- Sleep-related problems (apnea)
- Lowered tolerance to cold temperatures

This condition has been given the name of post-polio syndrome (PPS). While it is not considered life-threatening, PPS is emotionally devastating for many patients. It is a physically and emotionally painful reminder of what they once endured as children decades ago and may have to suffer through again. Fortunately, unlike polio, PPS is not contagious.

What causes PPS? No one is sure. Doctors suspect, however, that it is the result of years of wear and tear on the motor neurons that had to take over for the ones damaged during the first poliovirus infection. PPS does not usually begin to appear until at least fifteen years after the original onset of polio.

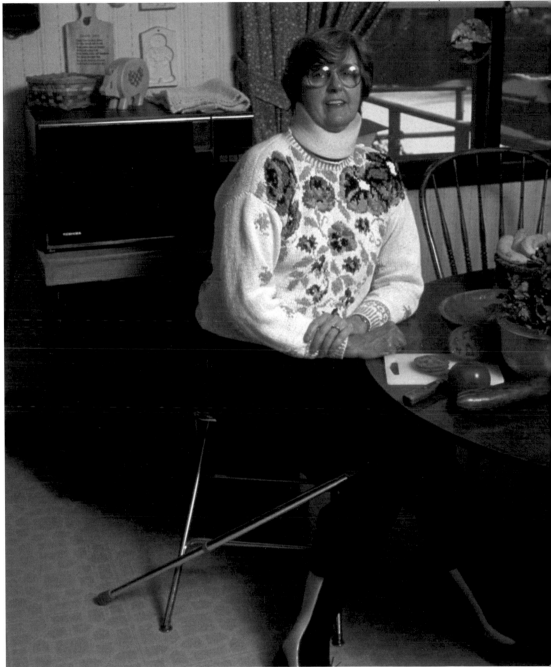

Decades after the original onset of polio, its symptoms of muscle weakness can return. PPS can even cause some patients to wear neck and/ or leg braces once again.

When its symptoms do begin to appear, PPS moves slowly. As time passes, the discomfort grows, and it becomes harder for the sufferer to perform normal daily activities.

The treatment for PPS involves little more than treating the most disturbing of its symptoms. Exercises are recommended for increasing muscle strength, and medications are given to help control pain and reduce fatigue. Counseling is often provided, since this new condition can bring back memories of a traumatic period in the patient's childhood.

In 1984, Dr. Laura Halstead, the director of the Post-Polio Program at the National Rehabilitation Hospital in Washington, D.C., organized the first international conference on the syndrome. The goals of the conference were to find ways to increase public awareness of the condition and raise funds for medical research. Since then, additional PPS conferences have been held in 1994 and 2000. Researchers are looking into the possibility of therapies related to nerve regrowth, but that is still years down the road. For now, PPS victims can do what they did long ago: band together, support research and testing for a cure, and cope the best they can through sheer grit, determination, and courage.

TEN GREAT QUESTIONS
to ask a DOCTOR

1 Has polio been eradicated worldwide?

2 Is there any chance I could become infected with the poliovirus in North America?

3 How is the virus spread, and how can you prevent spread and infection?

4 Can a vaccinated person with immunity to the poliovirus still be infected by it and, while remaining healthy, accidentally "carry" it to others who have not been vaccinated?

5 At what age should the polio vaccine first be administered, and when should follow-up vaccinations be given?

6 Is there any risk or danger associated with the polio vaccine?

7 Do some people fail to receive immunity from the vaccination?

8 Is there any risk or danger associated with not being vaccinated?

9 If I am traveling to one of the countries where the poliovirus is still "wild" and I have been vaccinated, what other precautions should I take, if any?

10 Where can my grandparent receive help for his or her symptoms of PPS?

GLOSSARY

amputate To cut off all or part of a limb of the body.

antibody A protein made by the immune system to respond to and fight infectious agents or foreign cells.

atmospheric pressure The pressure exerted by the earth's atmosphere at any given point.

atrophy A wasting away of a part of the body.

contagious Easily spread from person to person.

encephalitis An inflammation of the lining of the brain.

epidemic A new outbreak (i.e., beyond normal levels) of a disease that affects a population.

formaldehyde A colorless, toxic, water-soluble gas used in vaccine preparation to inactivate the poliovirus.

gastrointestinal Pertaining to the stomach and intestines.

humanitarian A person actively engaged in promoting human welfare and social reforms; characterized by a commitment to relieve suffering, deliver aid, and promote human health and welfare.

immune system The body's defenses that recognize and fight agents of infectious disease.

immunity The ability of an organism to resist, protect against, and/or fight infection.

indigenous Characteristic of a particular region or country.

orthopedist A doctor who deals with the prevention or correction of injuries and disorders of the skeletal system.

pediatrician A doctor who specializes in childhood diseases and the treating of children.

poliomyelitis The disease caused by infection with the poliovirus, which in some patients causes paralysis and even death; also known as polio.

quarantine A strict isolation imposed to prevent the spread of disease; the period of time when a contagious person is placed in isolation during a disease outbreak.

spasm An involuntary muscle contraction.

vaccination The practice of giving a foreign substance, such as a weakened form of a virus, to someone to generate immunity to an infectious agent.

virus A microscopic infectious agent that uses other living cells to replicate; many viruses cause disease.

FOR MORE INFORMATION

American Public Health Association
800 I Street NW
Washington, DC 20001
(202) 777-2742
Web site: http://www.apha.org
The American Public Health Association is an organi-
    zation of health professionals dedicated to improving
    public health.

Centers for Disease Control and Prevention
1600 Clifton Road
Atlanta, GA 30333
(800) 232-4636
Web site: http://www.cdc.gov
The Centers for Disease Control and Prevention is an
    organization that provides the public with reliable
    information about disease and health-related topics.

Global Polio Eradication Initiative
Avenue Appia 20
1211 Geneva 27
Switzerland
Web site: http://www.polioeradication.org
The goal of the Global Polio Eradication Initiative is
    to ensure that no child will ever again know the
    crippling effects of polio. It is the largest public
    health initiative the world has ever known.

Health Canada
A.L. 0904A
Ottawa, ON K1A 0K9
Canada
(613) 957-2991

Web site: http://www.hc-sc.gc.ca

Health Canada is a government department that helps
Canadians maintain and improve their health.

March of Dimes Foundation

1275 Mamaroneck Avenue

White Plains, NY 10605

(888) MODIMES (663-4637)

Web site: http://www.marchofdimes.com

The March of Dimes works to improve the health of babies
by preventing birth defects, premature birth, and infant
mortality. It carries out this mission through research,
community services, education, and advocacy to save
infants' lives. March of Dimes researchers, volunteers,
educators, outreach workers, and advocates work together
to give all babies a fighting chance against the threats to
their health: prematurity, birth defects, and low birth weight.

National Institute of Neurological Disorders and Stroke

P.O. Box 5801

Bethesda, MD 20824

(800) 352-9424

Web site: http://www.ninds.nih.gov

The mission of the National Institute of Neurological
Disorders and Stroke is to reduce the burden of neurological disease—a burden borne by every age group, by
every segment of society, by people all over the world.

National Institutes of Health (NIH)

9000 Rockville Pike

Bethesda, MD 20892

(301) 402-9612

Web site: http://www.nih.gov

The NIH's mission is science in pursuit of fundamental
   knowledge about the nature and behavior of living systems
   and the application of that knowledge to extend healthy
   life and reduce the burdens of illness and disability.

Post-Polio Project
National Rehabilitation Hospital (NRH)
102 Irving Street NW
Washington, DC 20010
(202) 877-1000
Web site: http://www.nrhrehab.org/Patient+Care/Programs+
   and+Service+Offerings/Outpatient+Services/Service_
   Page.aspx?id=39
Established in 1986, the NRH Post-Polio Program is the
   largest in the Washington metropolitan area and is one of
   only a few such programs across the country. Its goal is to
   help individuals become more effective in managing
   polio-related health problems through comprehensive
   evaluation, treatment, follow-up, and education. The
   program provides services to persons who had polio many
   years ago and now feel they are experiencing new health
   problems that may be related to polio.

Public Health Agency of Canada
1015 Arlington Street
Winnipeg, MB R3E3R2
Canada
(204) 789-2000
Web site: http://www.phac-aspc.gc.ca
The Public Health Agency of Canada is a government organization that promotes health and helps people prevent
   and control diseases, injuries, and infections.

United States Fund for the United Nations Children's Fund (UNICEF)
125 Maiden Lane, 11th Floor
New York, NY 10038
(212) 686-5522
Web site: http://www.unicef.org/index.php
UNICEF believes that nurturing and caring for children are the cornerstones of human progress. UNICEF was created with this purpose in mind—to work with others to overcome the obstacles that poverty, violence, disease, and discrimination place in a child's path.

World Health Organization (WHO)
Avenue Appia 20
1211 Geneva 27
Switzerland
Web site: http://www.who.int/en
The World Health Organization is part of the United Nations. It provides health leadership for the world and monitors health trends worldwide.

Web Sites

Due to the changing nature of Internet links, Rosen Publishing has developed an online list of Web sites related to the subject of this book. This site is updated regularly. Please use this link to access this list:

http://www.rosenlinks.com/epi/polio

FOR FURTHER READING

Aberth, John. *The First Horseman: Disease in Human History.* Upper Saddle River, NJ: Prentice Hall, 2006.

Arnold, Nick. *Deadly Diseases and Microscopic Monsters.* New York, NY: Scholastic, 2009.

Ballard, Carol. *Fighting Infectious Diseases.* Milwaukee, WI: World Almanac Library, 2007.

Bryn, Barnard. *Outbreak!: Plagues That Changed History.* New York, NY: Crown Books, 2005.

Claybourne, Anna. *World's Worst Germs: Microorganisms and Disease.* Chicago, IL: Heinemann-Raintree, 2005.

De la Bedoyere, Guy. *The First Polio Vaccine.* Strongsville, OH: Gareth Stevens, 2005.

Dobson, Mary J. *Disease: The Extraordinary Stories Behind History's Deadliest Killers.* London, England: Quercus Books, 2008.

Emmeluth, Donald. *Plague* (Deadly Diseases and Epidemics). New York, NY: Chelsea House Publications, 2005.

Farrell, Jeanette. *Invisible Enemies: Stories of Infectious Disease.* New York, NY: Farrar, Straus and Giroux, 2005.

Friedlander, Mark P., Jr. *Outbreak: Disease Detectives at Work* (Discovery!). Minneapolis, MN: Twenty-First Century Books, 2009.

Hostetter, Joyce Moyer. *Blue.* Honesdale, PA: Calkins Creek Books, 2006.

Hostetter, Joyce Moyer. *Comfort.* Honesdale, PA: Calkins Creek Books, 2009.

Kehret, Peg. *Small Steps: The Year I Got Polio.* Morton Grove, IL: Albert Whitman and Company, 2006.

Koch, Tom. *Cartographies of Disease: Maps, Mapping, and Medicine.* Redlands, CA: ESRI Press, 2005.

Krohn, Katherine. *Jonas Salk and the Polio Vaccine*.
　　Mankato, MN: Capstone Press, 2007.
Peters, Stephanie True. *The Battle Against Polio*. New York,
　　NY: Marshall Cavendish Books, 2005.
Sherman, Irwin W. *The Power of Plagues*. Washington, DC:
　　ASM Press, 2006.
Sherman, Irwin W. *Twelve Diseases That Changed Our World*.
　　Washington, DC: ASM Press, 2007.
Turkington, Carol, and Bonni Ashby. *Encyclopedia of
　　Infectious Diseases*. New York, NY: Facts on File, 2007.
Willett, Edward. *Disease-Hunting Scientist: Careers Hunting
　　Deadly Diseases* (Wild Science Careers). Berkeley
　　Heights, NJ: Enslow Publishers, 2009.

BIBLIOGRAPHY

Black, Kathryn. *In the Shadow of Polio: A Personal and Social History.* New York, NY: Da Capo Press, 1997.

Brinkley, Alan. *Franklin Delano Roosevelt.* New York, NY: Oxford University Press, 2009.

Bruno, Richard L. *The Polio Paradox: Understanding and Treating "Post-Polio Syndrome" and Chronic Fatigue.* New York, NY: Warner Books, 2003.

Bruno, Richard L. *The Polio Paradox: What You Need to Know.* New York, NY: Grand Central Publishing, 2002.

Finger, Anne. *Elegy for a Disease: A Personal and Cultural History of Polio.* New York, NY: St. Martin's Press, 2006.

Franklin D. Roosevelt Presidential Library and Museum. "Birthday Balls: Franklin D. Roosevelt and the March of Dimes." Retrieved August 2009 (http://docs.fdrlibrary.marist.edu/bdayb2.html).

Gould, Tony. *A Summer Plague: Polio and Its Survivors.* New Haven, CT: Yale University Press, 1997.

Kluger, Jeffrey. *Splendid Solution: Jonas Salk and the Conquest of Polio.* New York, NY: Berkley Books, 2006.

Lomazow, Steven, and Eric Fettman. *FDR's Deadly Secret.* New York, NY: PublicAffairs, 2010.

March of Dimes "Eddie Cantor and the Origin of the March of Dimes." May 2006. Retrieved August 2009 (http://www.marchofdimes.com/aboutus/20311_20401.asp).

Mayo Clinic Staff. "Polio." MayoClinic.com, March 2009. Retrieved August 2009 (http://www.mayoclinic/com/health/polio/DS00572/METHOD).

NIH Neurological Institute, Office of Communications and
    Public Liaison. "Post Polio Syndrome Resources Fact
    Sheet." 1998. Retrieved August 2009 (http://www.ppsr.
    com/ppsfactsheets.html).

Oshinsky, David M. *Polio: An American Story.* New York, NY:
    Oxford University Press, 2006.

Roberts, M. B. "Rudolph Ran and the World Went Wild."
    EPSN.com, 2007. Retrieved August 2009 (http://
    espn.go.com/sportscentury/features/
    00016444.html).

Rogers, Naomi. *Dirt and Disease: Polio Before FDR.* New
    Brunswick, NJ: Rutgers University Press, 1992.

Salgado, Sebastiao. *The End of Polio: A Global Effort to End
    a Disease.* New York, NY: Bulfinch Press, 2003.

Sass, Edmund J., with George Gottfried and Anthony Sorem.
    Polio's Legacy: An Oral History. Lanham, MD: University
    Press of America, 1996.

Shell, Marc. *Polio and Its Aftermath: The Paralysis
    of Culture.* Cambridge, MA: Harvard University
    Press, 2005.

Shreve, Susan Richards. *Warm Springs: Traces of a
    Childhood at FDR's Polio Haven.* New York, NY: Mariner
    Books, 2008.

Silver, Julie K. *Post-Polio Syndrome: A Guide for Polio
    Survivors and Their Families.* New Haven, CT: Yale
    University Press, 2002.

Smith, Jean Edward. *FDR.* New York, NY: Random
    House, 2008.

Smithsonian/National Museum of American History. "The
    American Epidemics: What Happened in the Polio
    Epidemics?" Retrieved August 2009 (http://americanhis-
    tory.si.edu/polio/americanepi/index.htm).

Time. "Medicine: Sister Kenny Endorsed." December 15, 1941. Retrieved August 2009 (http://www.time.com/time/magazine/article/0,9171,772865,00.html).

Wilson, Daniel J. *Living with Polio: The Epidemic and Its Survivors*. Chicago, IL: University of Chicago Press, 2007.

Wilson, Daniel J. *Polio* (Biographies of a Disease). Santa Barbara, CA: Greenwood, 2009.

World Health Organization. "Poliomyelitis." January 2008. Retrieved August 2009 (http://www.who.int/mediacentre/factsheets/fs114/en/index.html).

INDEX

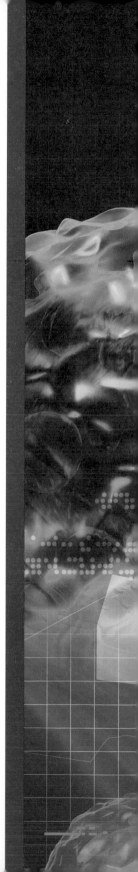

About the Author

Tamra B. Orr is the author of dozens of books for young readers, including many titles relating to science, medicine, health, disease, and society. She has won several awards for her books. Orr loves being an author because it gives her a chance to learn more about the world every day. She lives in the Pacific Northwest with her husband, children, cat, and dog. She makes sure her children have read every single one of her books.

Photo Credits

Designer: Sam Zavieh; Photo Researcher: Peter Tomlinson